MILES J DOLOR

Emergency Nursing Made Simple - Key Practices for Quick Expertise Without Overwhelming

A Must-Have Guide for Essential Skills and Techniques for ER Nurses.

First edition

This book was professionally typeset on Reedsy.
Find out more at reedsy.com

Contents

1

Vision for the Book

T his book is the ultimate resource for ER nurses. It equips them with the necessary skills and techniques to become experts in their field. It focuses on critical practices and strategies that enable nurses to develop their expertise quickly and effectively without feeling overwhelmed.

Whether you're a nursing student, a new graduate, or an experienced nurse, this book is a must-have resource for improving your emergency nursing skills. Nurse educators and healthcare professionals involved in emergency care will also find it highly beneficial.

By reading this book, you can access comprehensive and informative content that can help your professional development. You'll enhance your ability to provide high-quality care to your patients. With this essential guide, it's time to take your emergency nursing skills to the next level.

"Emergency Nursing Made Simple": Key Practices for Quick Expertise Without Overwhelming:

A Must-Have Guide for Essential Skills and Techniques for ER Nurses.

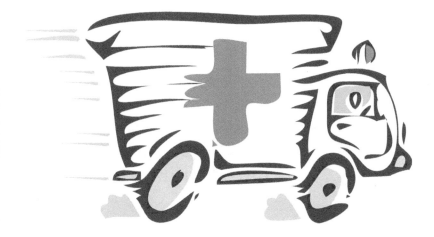

Introduction

Have you ever wondered what it's like to be an emergency nurse? Let me tell you, it's not an easy job. Janice is currently navigating the emergency room with her heart pounding, knowing that every decision she makes can be a matter of life and death. Emergency nursing is a fast-paced, demanding, and highly rewarding field that requires expertise and skill. It can be a challenging and stressful environment, but the profound sense of accomplishment that comes from helping others in their time of need makes it all worth it.

If you're looking for a guide to help you navigate the complexities of emergency nursing with confidence and ease, look no further! "Emergency Nursing Made Simple: Key Practices for Quick Expertise Without Overwhelming" is the book for you. It's not like any other book out there - it's unique in its approach to simplifying the dynamic field of emergency nursing, and it's bound to ignite your curiosity.

As the author, I aim to empower you with the essential abilities and methods to thrive in this fast-paced field, even with a busy schedule.

This book is a journey into the intricacies of emergency nursing, unveiling practical, vital practices that will revolutionize your approach to patient care.

Whether you're a seasoned ER nurse looking to enhance your skills or a new nurse eager to explore the field of emergency care, I'm here to assist and guide you. So, let's embark on this journey together and discover how we can simplify emergency nursing, one practice at a time!

4

Exploring the Fundamentals of Emergency Nursing

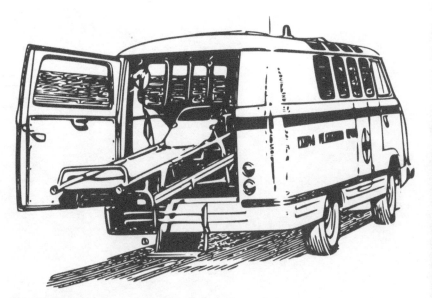

What is the Emergency Room?

The Emergency Room (ER), or the Emergency Department (ED), is a specialized unit within hospitals or healthcare centers that offers immediate medical attention to patients experiencing acute medical conditions or injuries. Operating 24/7, the ER provides swift medical aid to address medical emergencies, delivering constant support and care to ensure that help is always available when needed.

The ER is manned by a highly skilled and dedicated multidisciplinary team of healthcare professionals, including emergency physicians, nurses, paramedics, and various specialists, depending on the nature of the emergency. This team, driven by their commitment and proficiency, ensures that the primary objective of the ER is met—to stabilize patients and address their immediate medical needs to prevent further complications.

The Emergency Room (ER) is a crucial component of the healthcare system, serving as the first point of contact for patients who experience medical emergencies. Equipped with state-of-the-art medical equipment and technology, the ER enables healthcare professionals to diagnose and treat patients promptly and accurately. In a medical emergency, it is imperative to seek medical attention immediately, and the ER provides the necessary care to ensure the best possible outcomes.

To summarize, the ER is an essential element of the healthcare system, providing urgent medical care to patients in need. The highly skilled and dedicated team of healthcare professionals in the ER work tirelessly to stabilize patients and address their immediate medical needs, ensuring that patients receive the best possible outcomes when requiring immediate medical attention.

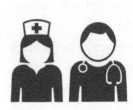 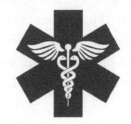 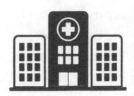

What is Emergency Nursing?

Did you know that emergency nursing, or emergency room nursing, is a super important nursing field? ER nurses specialize in providing timely and comprehensive care to patients experiencing acute medical conditions or injuries in the emergency department (ED) of hospitals or healthcare facilities. They are critical in assessing, prioritizing, and managing patients who come to the ED needing immediate medical attention. ER nurses are superheroes who work tirelessly to ensure patients are provided with the best possible care and treatment to improve their health outcomes. So, next time you're in the ED, be sure to give your ER nurse a big thank you for all that they do!

History

Over time, emergency nursing has evolved to adapt to the changing requirements of healthcare systems and advancements in medical technology. The significant changes that have taken place in healthcare systems and medical technology have impacted emergency nursing significantly. The roots of emergency nursing can be traced back to the early 1900s when nurses started to specialize in providing care for acutely ill and injured patients in hospital emergency departments. In the beginning, emergency nursing primarily involved triage and primary patient care. However, as emergency departments became more complex and specialized, emergency nurses' roles expanded to include diverse clinical skills and responsibilities.

Scope of Practice

Emergency nursing is all about caring for people going through tough times with their health. Emergency nurses are superheroes who help patients with acute illnesses, injuries, and medical emergencies. They work in various settings, like hospital emergency departments, trauma centers, urgent care clinics, and pre-hospital emergency services. The incredible individuals collaborate with other healthcare experts to guarantee that patients receive top-notch care. If you're ever in an emergency, these are the people you want on your side.

Their scope of practice may include:

1. **Triage**: Prioritizing patient care based on the severity of their condition and ensuring that those with life-threatening emergencies receive prompt attention.
2. **Assessment**: Conducting comprehensive assessments of patients, including obtaining medical histories, performing physical examinations, and monitoring vital signs.
3. **Treatment**: Administer medications, perform medical procedures, and provide interventions to stabilize patients and address their immediate medical needs.
4. **Patient Advocacy**: Advocating for patients' needs, ensuring their safety, and promoting their well-being throughout their ED stay.
5. **Collaboration**: Collaborating with physicians, other healthcare

professionals, and support staff to coordinate patient care and facilitate efficient workflow in the ED.

6. **Patient Education**: Providing information to patients and their families regarding their medical conditions, treatment plans, and discharge instructions to enhance comprehension and compliance with care plans.

7. **Crisis Management**: Responding effectively to medical emergencies, trauma cases, and other critical situations with composure and competence.

8. **Documentation**: Adhere to legal and regulatory guidelines for keeping precise and comprehensive patient assessments, interventions, and results records.

Nurses working in emergency situations require specialized expertise, critical thinking abilities, and effective decision-making skills to operate efficiently in a fast-paced and ever-changing environment. They must be adaptable, resourceful, and empathetic, as they frequently encounter patients facing life-threatening situations or experiencing extreme distress.

Role of Emergency Nurses within the Healthcare System

Emergency nurses, as the backbone of our healthcare system, play a unique and invaluable role that often goes unnoticed. They are the first responders to patients with acute and potentially life-threatening conditions, demonstrating exceptional skills in triaging, assessing, and initiating appropriate interventions to stabilize patients. Their hard work and dedication to advocating for evidence-based practices, maintaining high standards of quality and professionalism, and ensuring patient safety and well-being are truly awe-inspiring.

Emergency nurses, with their tireless efforts, significantly improve healthcare service standards, driven by their unwavering commitment to providing specialized care during times of crisis. Their competence, compassion, and dedication profoundly impact the outcomes of patients and their loved ones during critical moments. The selfless service and inspirational work of emergency nurses make them an irreplaceable asset to our healthcare system, and their efforts are crucial to achieving favorable results and ensuring that patients receive the best possible care.

Fundamental Concepts in Emergency Nursing

1. Patient Assessment:

- Conducting thorough and systematic assessments of patients is crucial in emergency nursing to identify life-threatening conditions and prioritize care.
- Assessments include obtaining medical histories, performing physical examinations, and monitoring vital signs to gather relevant information about the patient's condition.

2. Critical Thinking:

- Emergency nurses must possess strong critical thinking skills to rapidly analyze information, recognize patterns, and make informed decisions in high-pressure situations.
- They must be able to assess the severity of patients' conditions quickly, anticipate potential complications, and determine appropriate interventions.

3. Prioritization:

- Prioritizing patient care is essential in the fast-paced emergency department (ED) environment, where multiple patients with varying degrees of urgency may require attention simultaneously.
- Nurses use triage systems, such as the Emergency Severity Index (ESI), to prioritize patients based on the severity of their conditions and allocate resources effectively.

4. Communication Skills:

- Effective communication is vital in emergency nursing for conveying critical information to patients, families, and healthcare team members.
- Nurses must communicate concisely and compassionately, especially during stressful situations, to ensure accurate understanding and facilitate collaborative decision-making.

Importance of Quick Decision-Making and Adaptability:

1. Quick Decision-Making:

- Emergency nurses often face time-sensitive situations requiring immediate action to save lives or prevent further deterioration.
- Rapid decision-making skills allow nurses to prioritize interventions, initiate treatments, and promptly escalate care to address emergent patient needs.

2. Adaptability:

- The emergency department environment is dynamic and unpredictable, requiring nurses to adapt quickly to changing circumstances and patient needs.

• Nurses must be flexible and resourceful, able to adjust their approach to patient care based on evolving priorities, available resources, and new information.

Excellent patient assessment, critical thinking, prioritization, and communication skills are essential in emergency nursing. Given the challenging and fast-paced environment, nurses need these skills to provide high-quality care. Quick decision-making and adaptability are critical attributes that enable nurses to respond effectively to emergent situations and optimize patient outcomes. By mastering these fundamental concepts and embracing the demands of the ER environment, emergency nurses can excel in their roles and make a significant difference in the lives of those they serve.

5

Mastering Essential Skills for Effective Patient Care

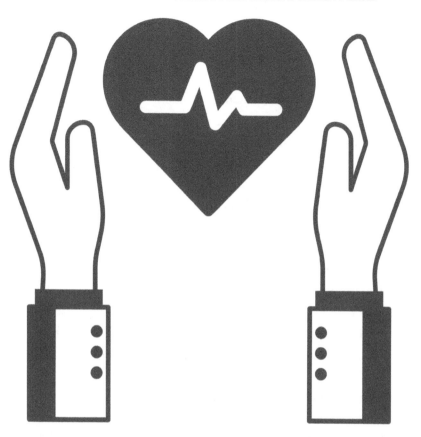

P atient Assessment Skills

The competency to accurately assess patients is a crucial skill required in the healthcare industry. It involves evaluating, analyzing, and interpreting information to understand the patient's condition, symptoms, and overall health status. By conducting a comprehensive patient assessment, healthcare professionals can develop effective treatment plans that address patients' needs and improve their health outcomes. Therefore, having strong patient assessment skills is essential for healthcare providers to provide quality care and ensure positive patient outcomes.

1. Obtaining Medical Histories:

- **Communication**: Establish rapport with the patient and obtain relevant medical history information by asking open-ended questions and actively listening to their responses.
- **Prioritization**: Identify critical aspects of the medical history, such as pre-existing conditions, allergies, medications, and recent illnesses or injuries, to assess the patient's baseline health status and potential risk factors.
- **Documentation**: Accurately document the patient's medical history, including chief complaints, past medical/surgical history, medications, allergies, immunization status, and social history, to facilitate continuity of care and inform subsequent interventions.

2. Performing Physical Examinations:

- **Systematic Approach**: Conduct a comprehensive head-to-toe physical examination using a systematic approach to ensure all body systems are assessed thoroughly.
- **Observation**: Observe the patient's general appearance, level of consciousness, skin color, and vital signs to gather initial information about their overall condition and identify any immediate concerns.
- **Assessment Techniques**: Utilize appropriate assessment techniques, such as inspection, palpation, percussion, and auscultation, to assess each body system systematically and identify abnormalities or signs of injury or illness.
- **Special Considerations**: Pay attention to specific assessment

considerations relevant to emergency nursing, such as assessing for signs of trauma, neurological deficits, respiratory distress, cardiovascular instability, or abdominal pain.

3. Interpreting Vital Signs:

- **Monitoring**: Continuously monitor and interpret vital signs, including temperature, heart rate, blood pressure, respiratory rate, and oxygen saturation, to assess the patient's physiological status and identify signs of instability or deterioration.
- **Baseline Comparison**: Compare current vital signs to the patient's baseline values (if available) and age-specific norms to identify deviations that may indicate changes in the patient's condition.
- **Trends Analysis**: Evaluate trends in vital signs over time to assess the patient's response to interventions, detect early signs of deterioration, and guide ongoing management decisions.
- **Critical Thinking**: Integrate vital sign data with other assessment findings and clinical context to comprehensively understand the patient's condition and prioritize interventions accordingly.

Conducting thorough patient assessments in the emergency setting requires communication skills, clinical knowledge, and critical thinking abilities. By obtaining comprehensive medical histories, performing systematic physical examinations, and accurately interpreting vital signs, emergency nurses can gather essential information to guide clinical decision-making and provide optimal care to patients who need help.

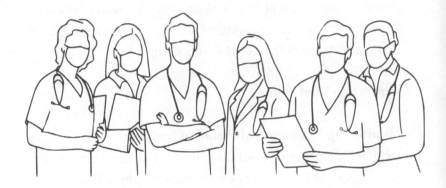

ER Nursing Assignments

In the emergency department (ED), nurses are the compassionate caregivers who provide prompt and effective care to needy patients. Their role is vital in ensuring patients receive the care they require during difficult times. Nurses understand the importance of providing comfort and support to patients experiencing medical emergencies and are dedicated to making a difference in their lives. They are assigned various roles based on their expertise and the needs of the patients. Some common ER nurse assignments and their specific roles include:

Triage Nurse:

- Role: Assess and prioritize patients based on the severity of their condition.
- Responsibilities: Conduct initial assessments, gather vital signs, determine the urgency of care, and ensure patients with life-threatening conditions receive immediate attention.

Primary Nurse:

- Role: Coordinate and manage assigned patients' care throughout their ED stay.
- Responsibilities: Conduct detailed assessments, develop and implement care plans, administer treatments, monitor patient progress, communicate with the healthcare team, and advocate for patients' needs.

Charge Nurse:

- Role: Oversee the operations of the ED during their shift and provide leadership to the nursing staff.
- Responsibilities: Coordinate patient flow, assign tasks to nurses, ensure adherence to protocols and policies, address any issues or concerns, serve as a resource for staff and patients, and maintain efficiency and safety within the ED.

Trauma Nurse:

- Role: Provide specialized care to patients with traumatic injuries or conditions.
- Responsibilities: Assess and stabilize trauma patients, administer emergency interventions, coordinate with other healthcare professionals, and ensure timely and appropriate care for trauma patients.

Critical Care Nurse:

- Role: Provide intensive care to critically ill or unstable patients in the ED.
- Responsibilities: Monitor patients' vital signs and condition, administer medications and treatments, perform advanced interventions such as intubation or defibrillation, collaborate with other health-

care providers, and ensure optimal care for critically ill patients.

Fast Track Nurse:

- Role: Provide rapid assessment and treatment to patients with minor injuries or illnesses.
- Responsibilities: Conduct quick assessments, administer essential treatments and medications, perform minor procedures, provide patient education, and facilitate timely discharge or referral for patients with less urgent conditions.

The tasks assigned to emergency department nurses may vary depending on the size of the department, the resources available, and the unique needs of the patients being treated. Moreover, nurses in the emergency department often work as a team to ensure that the care provided is thorough and efficient.

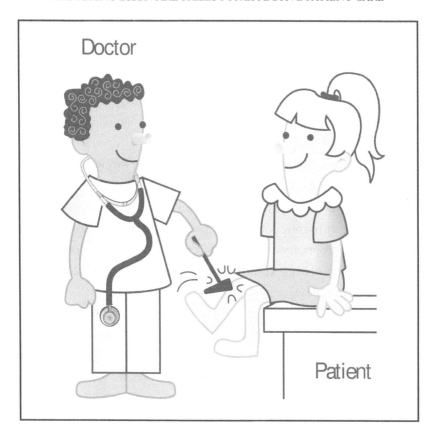

Common Emergency Procedures Performed by ER Nurses

In an emergency room, nurses are trained to perform a range of emergency procedures to stabilize and treat patients who arrive with acute medical conditions or injuries. Some standard emergency procedures ER nurses perform include administering medication, monitoring vital signs, performing CPR, managing bleeding, managing the airway, and providing wound care. These procedures require quick thinking, sound judgment, and excellent communication skills.

1. Wound Care:

- **Step-by-Step Instructions**:

1. Put on personal protective equipment (PPE), including gloves and, if needed, a mask and gown.
2. Assess the wound for size, depth, presence of foreign objects, and signs of infection.
3. Using a gentle irrigation technique, clean the wound with sterile saline or antiseptic solution, removing all debris and bacteria.
4. Apply appropriate wound dressings based on the type and severity of the wound (e.g., sterile gauze, non-adherent bandages, hydro-colloid dressings).
5. Use adhesive tape or bandages to fix the dressing and ensure it's not too tight and does not affect blood circulation.
6. Provide instructions to the patient for wound care at home, including signs of infection and when to seek medical attention.

Safety Considerations:

- Use proper infection control measures to prevent cross-contamination.
- Be cautious when handling sharp objects or contaminated materials to avoid accidental injuries.
- Ensure adequate pain management for the patient during wound care procedures.

2. Splinting:

- **Step-by-Step Instructions**:

1. Assess the injured limb for deformity, swelling, and tenderness, and immobilize the joint above and below the suspected fracture site.
2. Prepare the splinting materials, such as pads, elastic bandages, or commercial splints.
3. Apply padding to protect bony prominence and reduce pressure points.
4. Place the splint along the injured limb, ensuring proper alignment and immobilization of the fracture.
5. Use elastic bandages or Velcro straps to secure the splint, ensuring it is not too tight to affect the circulation but snug enough to stay in place.
6. Reassess neurovascular status distal to the splint to ensure adequate circulation and sensation.

Safety Considerations:

- Avoid excessive pressure or constriction when splinting to prevent complications such as compartment syndrome.
- Monitor the patient closely for signs of neurovascular compromise, such as numbness, tingling, or coolness distal to the splint.

3. **IV Insertion**:

- **Step-by-Step Instructions**:

1. Verify the patient's identity and assess for contraindications to IV access (e.g., allergies, medical conditions, previous complications).
2. Choose an appropriate site for IV insertion, typically the veins of the arms or hands, using a tourniquet to engorge the vein.
3. Cleanse the selected site with an antiseptic solution and allow it to

dry completely.

4. A sterile IV catheter and securement device should be used to insert the catheter into the vein at a 15-30 degree angle, advancing the catheter until blood return is observed.

5. Stabilize and secure the catheter with adhesive dressing or transparent film.

6. Flush the catheter with saline solution to confirm patency and secure the IV tubing to the catheter hub.

Safety Considerations:

• Use an aseptic technique to prevent bloodstream infections and other complications.

• Ensure proper catheter size selection to minimize the risk of infiltration or phlebitis.

• Monitor the IV site regularly for signs of complications such as swelling, redness, or pain.

4. **Medication Administration**:

• **Step-by-Step Instructions**:

1. Verify the patient's identity and confirm the medication order with the prescriber, checking for allergies and contraindications.

2. Prepare the medication according to institutional policies and manufacturer guidelines, verifying the correct medication, dose, route, and administration technique.

3. Choose an appropriate site for medication administration based on the medication's compatibility and patient preference (e.g., IV, oral, subcutaneous, intramuscular).

4. Administer the medication using the prescribed route and tech-

nique, ensuring accurate dosage and timing.

5. Monitor the patient for adverse reactions or unwanted effects after giving medication.
6. Document the medication administration, including the medication name, dose, route, time, and patient response.

Safety Considerations:

- Double-check medication calculations and administration techniques to prevent medication errors.
- Educate the patient about the purpose, potential side effects, and administration instructions for the prescribed medication.
- Monitor the patient closely for signs of adverse reactions or complications during and after medication administration.

Proficiency, attention to detail, and strict adherence to safety protocols are critical when performing standard emergency procedures in the ER. By following step-by-step instructions and considering safety considerations, ER nurses can effectively manage wounds, splints, IV insertions, and medication to provide optimal patient care in emergencies.

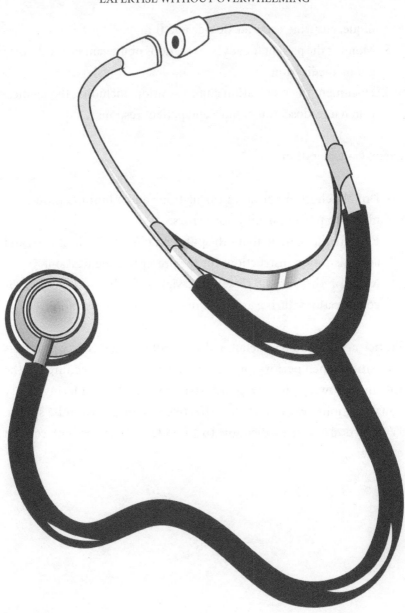

Principles of Triage and Prioritization in the ED

Triage is an essential procedure in the emergency room that involves systematically assessing patients and categorizing them based on the severity of their condition. This process helps prioritize patients according to their care needs, allowing for the efficient allocation of limited resources. The primary goal of triage is to ensure that patients receive timely and appropriate interventions that align with their clinical requirements. The triage process is guided by several fundamental principles.

1. **Urgency Assessment**: Triage nurses systematically and accurately assess patients' conditions. This assessment includes evaluating vital signs, symptoms, medical history, and chief complaints to determine the level of urgency.
2. **Triage Scales**: Various triage scales, such as the Emergency Severity Index (ESI), Manchester Triage System (MTS), and Canadian Triage and Acuity Scale (CTAS), are used to categorize patients into different priority levels depending on the seriousness of their ailment. These scales often employ color-coded categories (e.g., red for immediate, yellow for urgent, green for non-urgent) to denote the urgent care required.
3. **Algorithmic Approach**: Triage nurses follow established algorithms or protocols to guide their decision-making process. These algorithms consider specific criteria (e.g., vital signs, symptoms, trauma mechanism) to assign patients to the appropriate triage category.
4. **Continuous Reassessment**: Triage is not a one-time process; it requires ongoing reassessment of patients' conditions to identify changes in status or new priorities. Nurses must monitor patients closely and adjust their triage decisions to ensure that the most

critical cases receive timely attention.

5. **Team Collaboration**: Effective triage relies on collaboration among healthcare team members, including nurses, physicians, and ancillary staff. Communication and coordination are essential to ensure patients are triaged promptly and receive appropriate interventions based on their priority level.

6. **Ethical Considerations**: Triage decisions may involve complex ethical dilemmas, such as allocating resources during mass casualty incidents or prioritizing care for critically ill patients. Nurses must adhere to ethical principles like fairness, justice, and beneficence while making triage decisions in challenging circumstances.

7. **Documentation**: Accurate documentation of triage assessments, priority assignments, and interventions is essential for continuity of care, communication among healthcare providers, and legal purposes. Nurses must document pertinent information in the patient's medical record according to institutional policies and regulatory requirements.

By implementing these principles, triage nurses can prioritize patient care in the emergency department. This helps ensure that critical cases are given prompt attention while optimizing resource utilization and patient outcomes. The ability to triage patients effectively is crucial for managing patient flow, reducing wait times, and delivering timely interventions to those who need them most.

What is the Emergency Severity Index (ESI) Triage System?

Hospitals worldwide have implemented a system called the Emergency Severity Index (ESI) to help classify patients based on the severity of their condition. This system allows the emergency department (ED) to determine the level of resources required to provide the best possible care for each patient. The ESI system is a widely used triage system in EDs that classifies patients into one of five levels. The goal of this system is to prioritize patients efficiently and ensure that everyone receives the care they need. It guarantees that patients with the most critical needs get prompt attention while optimizing patient resources.

ESI Triage Levels:

1. **ESI Level 1 (Immediate)**: Patients in this category require immediate attention due to life-threatening conditions or critical injuries. Examples include cardiac arrest, severe trauma, or respiratory distress. These patients often need rapid resuscitation and intensive interventions.
2. **ESI Level 2 (Emergent)**: This category includes patients with potentially serious conditions that require prompt evaluation and treatment. Examples include chest pain suggestive of a heart attack, stroke symptoms, or severe pain uncontrolled by medication. These patients may need diagnostic tests or interventions within a short timeframe.
3. **ESI Level 3 (Urgent)**: Patients in this category have urgent but not immediately life-threatening conditions. Examples include minor trauma, uncomplicated fractures, or exacerbations of chronic illnesses. While these patients require timely care, their conditions are stable enough to wait briefly for evaluation and treatment.
4. **ESI Level 4 (Less Urgent)**: Patients with non-urgent conditions or minor injuries are assigned to this category. Examples include minor lacerations, sprains, or minor infections. These patients can safely wait for evaluation and treatment without compromising their health.
5. **ESI Level 5 (Non-urgent)**: Patients with non-urgent complaints or minor ailments fall into this category. Examples include medi-

cation refills, minor cold symptoms, or non-specific complaints without significant symptoms. These patients can typically wait longer for evaluation and may not require immediate medical attention.

Application of ESI Triage Criteria:

Example 1:

In the emergency department, a male patient who is 55 years old has arrived with sudden onset chest pain radiating to his left arm and shortness of breath. He appears diaphoretic and is in significant distress. Upon assessment, his vital signs reveal tachycardia, hypotension, and an oxygen saturation of 88% on room air. Based on these findings, the patient is triaged as ESI Level 1 (Immediate) due to the high likelihood of a myocardial infarction or other life-threatening cardiac event requiring immediate intervention.

Example 2:

A 25-year-old female arrives at the ED with a deep laceration on her forearm sustained while cooking. Pressure was applied to control the bleeding, and the patient's vital signs were normal while remaining hemodynamically stable. The laceration appears clean and does not involve any underlying structures. Based on the absence of significant bleeding and stable vital signs, the patient is triaged as ESI Level 3 (Urgent) for prompt evaluation and wound closure to prevent infection and optimize wound healing.

These examples demonstrate how the ESI triage system can effectively prioritize patient care based on the acuity of their conditions, ensuring that those with the most critical needs receive timely interventions while balancing resource allocation for all patients in the ED.

What is ER-Focused Assessment?

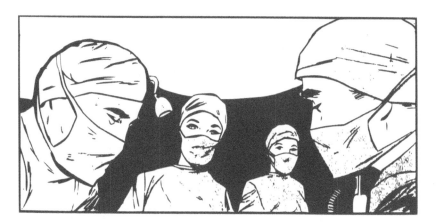

Did you know that healthcare professionals in emergency departments systematically evaluate and prioritize patients based on their presenting complaints or conditions? This is called the Emergency Room (ER) Focused Assessment, and it's a helpful way to gather essential information quickly through a targeted examination. The aim is to identify potential life-threatening issues and determine the appropriate action.

Critical components of an ER Focused Assessment may include:

1. **Chief Complaint**: Identifying the primary reason for the patient's visit to the emergency department.
2. **History of Present Illness (HPI)**: Obtaining a concise and

relevant history of the current symptoms or injury, including onset, duration, exacerbating or relieving factors, and associated symptoms.

3. **Vital Signs**: Assessing vital signs such as blood pressure, heart rate, respiratory rate, temperature, and oxygen saturation to gauge the patient's overall physiological status.

4. **Focused Physical Examination**: Conducting a targeted physical examination focused on the areas relevant to the patient's chief complaint or presenting symptoms. This may involve assessing specific body systems or regions based on the nature of the illness or injury.

5. **Diagnostic Tests**: Ordering and interpreting diagnostic tests such as laboratory studies (e.g., blood tests, urine analysis), imaging studies (e.g., X-rays, CT scans), or other specialized tests to evaluate the patient's condition further.

6. **Pain Assessment**: Evaluating the patient's pain level using standardized pain assessment tools and providing appropriate pain management interventions as needed.

7. **Risk Assessment**: Identify any potential risks or complications associated with the patient's condition and take proactive measures to mitigate these risks.

8. **Disposition Planning**: Determining the appropriate disposition for the patient, which may include discharge home, admission to the hospital, referral to specialty services, or transfer to another facility for higher-level care.

The main objective of an assessment focused on emergency rooms is to evaluate patients and assess their level of urgency swiftly. This helps healthcare providers take prompt action and implement timely interventions, enhancing patient outcomes during emergencies.

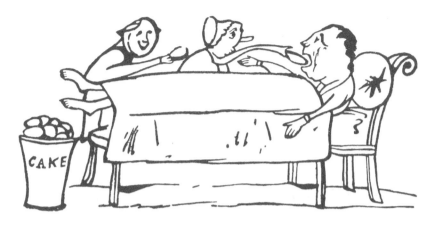

Standardized ER Protocol

Did you know that healthcare providers use standardized emergency room (ER) protocols to guide patient evaluation and initial management in the ER? These protocols are based on evidence-based guidelines and best practices in emergency medicine to provide efficient care. By streamlining and standardizing the process for common ER conditions, they ensure that nurses can initiate appropriate interventions promptly, even before a physician or advanced practice provider evaluates the patient.

The protocols involve steps or actions based on the patient's presenting symptoms, vital signs, and medical history. They may include diagnostic tests, medication administration, procedures, and specialist referrals. For instance, a protocol for chest pain may consist of orders for an electrocardiogram (ECG), aspirin administration, and vital signs monitoring.

The main objective of these protocols is to evaluate patients and swiftly assess their urgency level. This helps healthcare providers take prompt action and implement timely interventions, enhancing patient outcomes during emergencies.

Triage Protocols

Stroke Symptoms

- Emergency Departments (EDs) often activate "stroke alerts" to notify the entire department when a patient requires urgent care due to a possible stroke.
- The triage nurse initiates patient transport to the CT scanner within 10 minutes of arrival.
- Common stroke symptoms include facial droop, numbness on one side of the body, and difficulty speaking or understanding speech. One mnemonic to aid in stroke recognition is B.E. F.A.S.T.
- Stroke symptoms are typically assigned an acuity level of ESI level 2 unless the patient has limited responsiveness or cannot protect their airway, in which case they are assigned level 1.

Chest Pain

- Chest pain is one of the most common complaints in the ED and may be challenging to assess for severity and acuity.
- Patients presenting with chest pain should be given an ESI level of at least 3.
- A protocol is initiated for an EKG within 10 minutes of arrival.
- When triaging chest pain, the patient's level of distress, ambulatory status, cardiac history, and EKG findings are considered.

Abdominal Pain

- Abdominal pain typically requires two or more resources and is categorized as level 3.
- Warning signs such as hypotension, pallor, diaphoresis, fever, or a "ripping" description of pain may warrant an upgrade to level 2.
- These symptoms may indicate conditions such as an abdominal aortic aneurysm.

Shortness of Breath

- Shortness of breath typically warrants at least an ESI level 3, involving laboratory tests, X-rays, and possibly medication.
- Factors to consider include the patient's breathing work, use of accessory muscles, and oxygenation status.
- Immediate oxygen application is necessary if the patient's oxygen saturation is compromised, elevating the acuity to at least level 2.

Broken Bones

- Patients often visit the ED for X-rays to assess potential fractures following minor injuries.
- Most cases are classified as ESI level 4 (one resource), but visible deformities may require conscious sedation and pain medication, elevating the acuity to level 3.
- Further questioning by the triage nurse is necessary to determine the mechanism of injury and whether the patient requires a higher acuity level, particularly in severe trauma cases.

Other High-Risk Situations

Conditions such as testicular torsion, diabetic ketoacidosis (DKA), hyperglycemic hyperosmolar non-ketotic syndrome (HHNS), and urinary retention should be classified as ESI level 2 due to their potential severity and complexity.

6

Managing Critical Situations in the ER

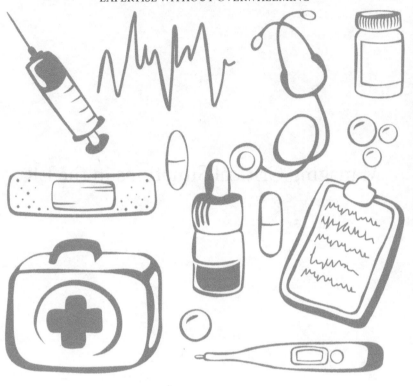

D id you know that emergency nurses play a vital role in providing immediate and effective care to patients during medical emergencies? Healthcare experts possess the necessary skills to deal with life-threatening scenarios, including cardiac arrest, trauma, and respiratory distress. They take charge of the problem and ensure that the required care is provided to those in need. By relying on various effective strategies and fulfilling their essential responsibilities, they help save lives and make a difference in their patients' lives.

1. Cardiac Arrest:

- Immediate Response: Emergency nurses are often the first responders to cardiac arrest situations. They initiate cardiopulmonary resuscitation (CPR) and coordinate the response team.
- Defibrillation: Nurses who are trained to deliver electrical shocks can operate defibrillators and restore the heart's normal rhythm..
- Medication Administration: They administer emergency medications such as epinephrine, amiodarone, or vasopressors as per the advanced cardiac life support (ACLS) guidelines.
- Documentation: Nurses accurately document the events, interventions performed, and patient responses for continuity of care.

2. Trauma:

- Primary Assessment: Nurses conduct rapid trauma assessments following the ABCDE (Airway, Breathing, Circulation, Disability, Exposure) approach to identify life-threatening injuries.
- Stabilization: They assist in stabilizing patients by controlling bleeding, immobilizing fractures, and managing airway and breathing.
- Diagnostic Procedures: Nurses may assist in performing diagnostic tests such as imaging studies or laboratory investigations to identify internal injuries.
- Coordination: The trauma team works with nurses, physicians, surgeons, and other healthcare professionals to guarantee that care is administered promptly and suitably.

3. Respiratory Distress:

- Assessment: Nurses assess respiratory status by monitoring oxygen saturation, respiratory rate, and breath sounds.

- Oxygen Therapy: They administer supplemental oxygen and titrate oxygen flow rates to maintain adequate oxygenation.
- Ventilator Management: Nurses may assist with mechanical ventilation, including ventilator setup, monitoring, and troubleshooting.
- Medication Administration: They administer bronchodilators, corticosteroids, or other respiratory medications as the physician prescribes.

Roles and Responsibilities of Emergency Nurses during Resuscitation

1. **Team Leader**: In many cases, the senior emergency nurse assumes the team leader role during resuscitation efforts. They coordinate team members, assign tasks, and ensure effective communication.
2. **Airway Management**: Nurses may be responsible for airway management, including positioning the patient, inserting airway adjuncts (e.g., oropharyngeal or nasopharyngeal airways), and assisting with endotracheal intubation.
3. **Medication Administration**: Nurses prepare and administer medications as directed by the physician, ensuring proper dosages, routes, and timing. They also monitor the patient's medication response and report any adverse reactions promptly.
4. **Documentation**: Nurses maintain accurate and detailed documentation of resuscitation events, including interventions performed, medications administered, and patient responses. This documentation is crucial for legal and quality assurance purposes.
5. **Support for Family and Loved Ones**: During resuscitation efforts, nurses provide emotional support and information to the patient's family and loved ones, keeping them informed about their condition and offering comfort during a distressing time.

The work of nurses in the emergency room is vital. They are adept at handling critical situations. Better healthcare practices can improve patient outcomes and raise survival rates.

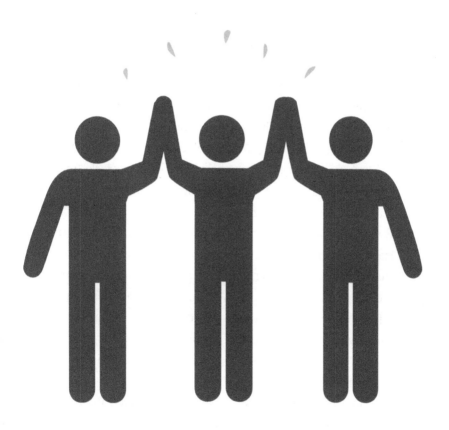

Importance of Collaboration and Teamwork in the ED

In an emergency department (ED), where time is of the essence and situations change rapidly, providing the best possible care to patients should be the top priority. However, this can only be achieved through effective teamwork and collaboration among healthcare providers. It is by working together that we can ensure optimal results for our patients. Therefore, it is crucial to prioritize collaboration to deliver exceptional patient care in the ED.

1. **Optimal Patient Outcome**s: By working collaboratively, healthcare providers can leverage their expertise to assess, diagnose, and treat patients more efficiently, leading to better outcomes and reduced morbidity and mortality rates.

2. **Efficient Resource Utilization**: Effective collaboration ensures that resources, including personnel, equipment, and facilities, are utilized efficiently. Team members can coordinate tasks, prioritize patient care, and streamline workflows to minimize delays and maximize resource utilization.

3. **Enhanced Patient Safety**: Collaboration reduces the risk of medical errors and adverse events by fostering open communication, shared decision-making, and mutual accountability among team members. This collaborative environment promotes a culture of safety and continuous quality improvement.

4. **Improved Staff Satisfaction**: A collaborative work environment fosters camaraderie, mutual respect, and professional growth among healthcare providers. Recognizing and valuing each other's contributions make team members feel supported and motivated, leading to higher job satisfaction and retention rates.

Effective Communication Techniques:

1. **Clear and Concise Communication**: Healthcare providers should communicate information clearly and concisely, using sim-

ple language and avoiding medical jargon. Clear communication ensures everyone understands the patient's condition, treatment plan, and assigned tasks.

2. **Active Listening**: Listening to colleagues' input, concerns, and suggestions promotes mutual understanding and effective collaboration. An environment of trust and respect can be established by fostering open expression of thoughts and relations among team members and acknowledging their perspectives.

3. **Closed-Loop Communication**: Implement closed-loop communication techniques to confirm that messages are accurately received and understood. This involves the sender delivering a statement, the receiver acknowledging receipt and understanding, and the sender confirming the receiver's acknowledgment.

4. **Structured Handoffs**: During shift changes or patient transfers, use structured handoff protocols (e.g., SBAR - Situation, Background, Assessment, Recommendation) to convey essential information systematically and comprehensively. This reduces the risk of information gaps and miscommunication.

Collaboration, effective communication, and interdisciplinary approaches are crucial for healthcare providers working in emergency departments to improve patient outcomes, promote safety, and foster a culture of teamwork and excellence. By utilizing unique skills and working together as a team, emergency departments can ensure patients receive the best care safely and efficiently. Adopting such an approach can help emergency departments to enhance patient care and establish a culture of excellence.

Crisis Management

A well-structured plan, clear protocols, and seamless coordination among healthcare providers are paramount when managing crises and emergencies in the emergency department (ED). Here is some guidance you can follow to help you effectively handle different types of crises and emergencies.

1. **Disaster Preparedness**:

- Develop Comprehensive Disaster Plans: Establish robust disaster plans that outline protocols for various types of disasters, such as natural disasters, infectious disease outbreaks, and mass casualty incidents. Collaborate with local emergency management agencies, community organizations, and other healthcare facilities to coordinate response efforts.
- Conduct Regular Drills and Exercises: Conduct regular disaster drills and tabletop exercises to test the effectiveness of disaster plans, identify areas for improvement, and familiarize staff with their roles and responsibilities during emergencies. Evaluate the response to each drill and incorporate lessons learned into future planning efforts.
- Stockpile Essential Supplies: Maintain adequate stockpiles of essential supplies, including medical supplies, medications, personal protective equipment (PPE), and emergency equipment. Regularly review and update inventory levels to ensure readiness for potential disasters.
- Establish Communication Protocols: Establish clear communication protocols to facilitate timely and accurate emergency communication. Utilize multiple communication channels, such as radios, mobile phones, and messaging systems, to ensure redundancy and resilience in communication networks.

2. Mass Casualty Incidents (MCIs):

- Activate MCI Protocols: Upon receiving notification of a mass casualty incident, activate MCI protocols to mobilize resources, triage patients, and coordinate response efforts. Designate a designated MCI command center to oversee operations and ensure effective communication and coordination.
- Implement Triage Systems: Implement triage systems, such as the

Simple Triage and Rapid Treatment (START) or the JumpSTART method, to prioritize patients based on the severity of their injuries and allocate resources accordingly. Train staff in triage protocols and ensure the availability of triage tags and equipment.

- Expand Treatment Capacity: Prepare to expand treatment capacity by establishing additional treatment areas, mobilizing additional staff, and utilizing alternate care sites if necessary. Implement surge capacity strategies to accommodate many patients while maintaining quality care standards.

- Coordinate with External Partners: Collaborate with external partners, such as EMS agencies, fire departments, law enforcement, and other healthcare facilities, to facilitate patient transport, resource allocation, and mutual aid support. Establish clear communication channels and designated liaison roles to streamline coordination efforts.

3. **Code Blue Responses**:

- Activate Code Blue Protocol: Upon identifying a patient in cardiac arrest or respiratory distress, activate the Code Blue protocol to initiate a rapid response team (RRT) response. Communicate the location of the emergency and provide relevant patient information to the RRT members.

- Perform High-Quality CPR: Ensure that healthcare providers perform high-quality cardiopulmonary resuscitation (CPR) according to established guidelines, including adequate chest compressions, proper airway management, and prompt defibrillation as indicated. Rotate compressors regularly to prevent fatigue and maintain effective CPR.

- Assign Roles and Responsibilities: Assign specific roles and responsibilities to team members during Code Blue responses, including

team leader, compressor, airway manager, medication adminis-
trator, and recorder. Clarify expectations and ensure each team
member understands and performs their role effectively.

• Conduct Post-Resuscitation Debriefings: Following a Code Blue
event, conduct post-resuscitation debriefings to review the response, identify areas for improvement, and provide emotional
support to team members. Encourage open discussion and feedback
to promote continuous learning and improvement.

What is a Rapid Sequence Intubation?

RSI is a specialized technique used in emergencies to secure a patient's
airway quickly. It involves administering sedatives and neuromuscular
blocking drugs to cause unconsciousness and paralysis, followed by
inserting an endotracheal tube into the trachea. Trained healthcare
providers perform RSI, and careful monitoring is required to ensure
patient safety. Plan, clear protocols, and seamless coordination among
healthcare providers are paramount when managing crises and emergencies in the emergency department (ED). Here is some guidance you
can follow to help you effectively handle different types of crises and
emergencies.

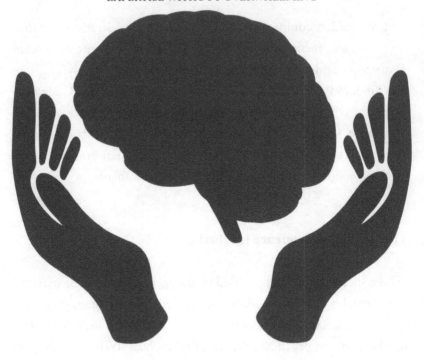

What is Code Stroke?

Did you know hospitals have a unique protocol called Code Stroke, which helps diagnose and treat suspected stroke patients faster? During a Code Stroke, a team of healthcare professionals, including emergency physicians, neurologists, radiologists, and nurses, works together to assess and manage the patient's condition quickly. It's crucial to recognize the signs of a stroke and to promptly seek medical attention if you suspect someone is experiencing one. Act fast to get help - it can make all the difference. Remember, every second counts! To help you remember the critical indicators of a stroke, you can use a helpful mnemonic called B.E. F.A.S.T.

- B is for Balance: Is there a loss of balance?
- E is for Eyes: Are the eyes clear and focused?
- F is for Face: Is there any asymmetry or drooping of the face?
- A is for Arm: Can both arms be moved freely?
- S is for Speech: Is there slurred speech or difficulty speaking?
- T is for Time: How long have these symptoms persisted? Act swiftly by calling 911 or heading to the ER is essential.

Emergency physicians are trained to conduct a **F.A.S.T.** exam for stroke assessment:

- F: Assess facial symmetry for any drooping.
- A: Evaluate arm mobility by asking the patient to raise both arms.
- S: Observe speech patterns for slurring or incoherence.
- T: Recognize the situation's urgency and seek immediate medical attention.

Recognizing the symptoms of a stroke and taking action immediately can significantly reduce its severity. It is vital to be aware of these signs to ensure timely intervention.

The protocol typically involves several critical steps:

1. **Rapid Assessment**: Medical personnel evaluate the patient promptly to assess symptoms and determine the likelihood of a stroke based on clinical signs, such as sudden-onset weakness, numbness, or difficulty speaking.
2. **Imaging Studies**: Urgent imaging studies, such as a computed tomography (CT) scan or magnetic resonance imaging (MRI), are performed to visualize the brain and identify any signs of stroke, such as ischemic or hemorrhagic lesions.

3. **Laboratory Tests**: Assessing different parameters, such as coagulation status and blood glucose levels, can provide additional information about the patient's condition, which may require blood tests.

4. **Treatment Initiation**: Once a stroke is confirmed, it is crucial to initiate appropriate medical interventions promptly. The outlined method can help reinstate blood flow to the impacted brain region and diminish further neurological harm. This may include administering clot-busting medications (thrombolytics) or performing interventional procedures such as thrombectomy.

5. **Continuous Monitoring**: The patient is closely monitored for any changes in neurological status or complications, and additional interventions are provided as needed to optimize outcomes.

The Code Stroke protocols are designed to streamline the diagnostic and treatment process, reduce treatment time, and improve patient outcomes. Acting quickly is crucial to minimize the long-term effects of stroke and prevent potential complications. It's critical to intervene early on to achieve the best possible results.

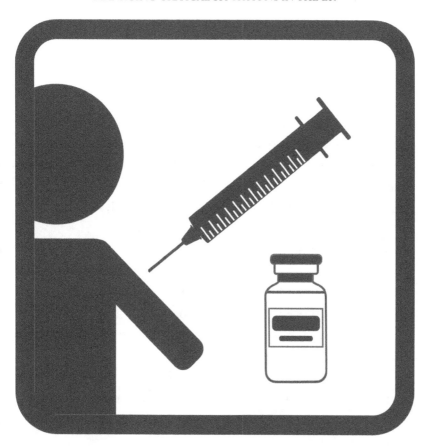

What is Sepsis Workup?

Sepsis is a medical condition that could be life-threatening if the body reacts negatively to an infection. Healthcare professionals use a systematic approach known as the sepsis workup protocol to manage sepsis efficiently. This protocol comprises several critical components that help healthcare providers identify the severity of sepsis and provide appropriate treatment. In this regard, let's look at the essential elements of the sepsis workup protocol that healthcare professionals follow to diagnose and treat sepsis effectively.

1. **Clinical Assessment**:

The first step is to complete the patient's clinical assessment. This process includes a thorough analysis of medical records, a physical check-up, and an evaluation of essential signs. Signs and symptoms suggestive of sepsis may include fever, elevated heart rate, rapid breathing, altered mental status, and signs of organ dysfunction.

2. **Diagnostic Tests**:

- Blood Cultures: Blood cultures are obtained to identify the causative pathogen(s) responsible for the infection. Cultures are typically drawn from multiple sites to increase the likelihood of detecting the infectious organism.
- Complete Blood Count (CBC): A CBC is performed to assess for leukocytosis (elevated white blood cell count), leukopenia (decreased white blood cell count), or abnormalities in other blood cell parameters.
- Serum Lactate Levels: Serum lactate levels are measured to assess tissue perfusion and identify patients at risk of septic shock. Elevated lactate levels may indicate tissue hypoperfusion and are associated with increased mortality in sepsis.
- Inflammatory Markers: Markers that cause inflammation, like C-reactive protein (CRP) and procalcitonin, can be evaluated to determine the intensity of the inflammatory response and assist in deciding the appropriate antibiotic treatment.
- Electrolyte and Renal Function Tests: Electrolyte levels, renal function tests (e.g., creatinine, blood urea nitrogen), and other metabolic parameters are evaluated to assess organ dysfunction

and guide fluid resuscitation.

3. **Imaging Studies**: Based on the clinical presentation and suspected source of infection, imaging studies like chest X-rays, abdominal ultrasound, or computed tomography (CT) scans may be required. These can help identify the source of infection and check for any complications, such as organ involvement or abscesses.

4. **Other Investigations**: Additional investigations may be indicated based on the patient's clinical presentation and suspected source of infection. This may include urine analysis and culture, sputum culture, wound swabs, or imaging of specific body regions.

5. **Treatment Initiation**: Prompt initiation of treatment is essential in sepsis management. This typically involves empirical broad-spectrum antibiotic therapy targeting the suspected pathogens based on the likely source of infection and local antimicrobial resistance patterns. Intravenous fluids may also be administered to optimize hemodynamic status and tissue perfusion.

6. **Monitoring and Reassessment**: Patients with sepsis require close monitoring of vital signs, hemodynamic parameters, and laboratory values to assess response to treatment and identify complications. Reassessment of clinical status and response to therapy guides ongoing management decisions, including adjustments to antibiotic therapy and fluid resuscitation.

The sepsis workup protocol enables healthcare providers to identify, diagnose, and treat sepsis. By following this protocol, healthcare professionals can proactively manage crises, improve patient outcomes, and reduce mortality. Adhering to these guidelines ensures that patients and staff remain safe and receive high-quality care during emergencies.

7

Building Confidence and Resilience in Emergency Situations

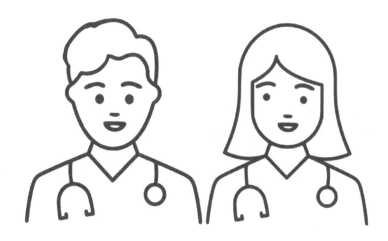

P rofessional Development

As an emergency nurse, focusing on professional development and career advancement is essential, which can help you excel in your field. To support you in this journey, here are some valuable tips and opportunities to help you enhance your skills, pursue specialization, obtain certifications, and engage in continuing education. These efforts will not only help you advance your career but also contribute to providing optimal patient care and outcomes.

1. Pursue Specialization:

- **Trauma Nursing**: Consider specializing in trauma nursing to provide specialized care to patients with traumatic injuries. Pursue opportunities to work in trauma centers or participate in trauma nursing courses and workshops to expand your knowledge and skills.
- **Critical Care Nursing**: Explore opportunities to specialize in critical care nursing, focusing on caring for critically ill or unstable patients. Obtain experience in intensive care units (ICUs) or pursue certifications such as the Critical Care Registered Nurse (CCRN) certificate to demonstrate your expertise in critical care nursing.
- **Pediatric Emergency Nursing**: If you are passionate about caring for pediatric patients, consider specializing in pediatric emergency nursing. Gain experience in pediatric emergency departments or certifications like the Certified Pediatric Emergency Nurse (CPEN) certification to improve your expertise in pediatric emergency care.

2. Obtain Certifications:

- **Certified Emergency Nurse (CEN)**: Consider obtaining the Certified Emergency Nurse (CEN) certification offered by the Board of Certification for Emergency Nursing (BCEN). This certification demonstrates your proficiency and competence in emergency nursing and can enhance your credibility and career prospects.

- **Advanced Certifications**: Explore advanced certifications such as the Certified Flight Registered Nurse (CFRN), Certified Emergency Nurse Practitioner (CENP), or Certified Pediatric Emergency Nurse (CPEN) to specialize further and advance your career in emergency nursing.

3. Engage in Continuing Education:

- **Attend Conferences and Workshops**: Attending emergency nursing conferences, workshops, and seminars is crucial for staying up-to-date with the latest trends and advancements in the field. These events also provide valuable opportunities for networking and professional development.
- **Enroll in Continuing Education Courses**: take advantage of continuing education courses and online learning modules tailored to emergency nursing practice. Topics may include trauma management, critical care nursing, disaster preparedness, and advanced life support techniques.
- **Seek Mentorship and Preceptorship**: Connect with experienced emergency nurses and seek mentorship and preceptorship opportunities to learn from their expertise and experience. Shadowing experienced nurses and engaging in hands-on learning can accelerate your professional development and confidence in emergency nursing practice.

4. Pursue Advanced Degrees:

- **Obtain Advanced Nursing Degrees**: If you're looking to further your career in emergency nursing leadership, education, or advanced practice roles, you may want to consider pursuing higher education. A Master of Science in Nursing (MSN) or a Doctor of

Nursing Practice (DNP) are examples of advanced degrees in the nursing field. This can expand your career opportunities in these areas.

- **Specialize in Nurse Practitioner Roles**: If you're interested in providing advanced diagnostic and treatment interventions in the emergency department, consider exploring opportunities to become a certified emergency nurse practitioner (ENP) or acute care nurse practitioner (ACNP).

Emergency nurses can advance their careers by specializing in a particular area, obtaining certifications, pursuing education, or obtaining advanced degrees. To maintain a healthy work-life balance, it is essential to prioritize self-care, which can help prevent burnout and manage stress. Simple steps like exercising regularly, eating well, getting enough sleep, seeking support, and pursuing relaxation can all contribute to better self-care and, in turn, better patient care.

Self-Care and Wellness

Emergency nurses can advance their careers by specializing in a particular area, obtaining certifications, pursuing education, or obtaining advanced degrees. Taking care of yourself is important for a healthy balance between work and personal life. This can help you avoid feeling overwhelmed and manage stress. Simple steps like exercising regularly, eating well, getting enough sleep, seeking support, and pursuing relaxation can all contribute to better self-care and, in turn, better patient care.

1. **Recognize the Importance of Self-Care**:

- Acknowledge that self-care is not selfish but essential for maintaining physical, mental, and emotional well-being.

- Understand that prioritizing self-care enables you to provide high-quality patient care and perform effectively as an emergency nurse.

2. **Implement Stress Management Techniques**:

- If you're feeling stressed, don't worry - there are things you can do to help you relax! Why not practice mindfulness and relaxation techniques like yoga, deep breathing, or meditation? They're great ways to reduce stress and promote relaxation.
- Regularly exercise to release tension, boost mood, and improve overall health.
- Take short breaks during shifts to decompress, recharge, and refocus your energy.

3. **Foster Supportive Relationships**:

- It is essential to build a network of supportive individuals, including colleagues, friends, and family members, who know the difficulties of working in emergency nursing and can offer emotional assistance.
- Participate in peer support groups or debriefing sessions to share experiences, seek advice, and process challenging situations.

4. **Set Boundaries and Prioritize Self-Care**:

- Establish clear boundaries between work and personal life to prevent burnout and maintain balance.
- Learn to say no to additional shifts or responsibilities when necessary to avoid overextending yourself.
- Schedule regular time off for rest, relaxation, and enjoyable activi-

ties outside of work.

5. Practice Healthy Lifestyle Habits:

- To ensure your energy levels, immune function, and overall health are supported, it's essential to maintain a diet that is balanced and contains nutritious foods.
- Good sleep is crucial, and a regular sleeping routine can maximize the benefits of rejuvenating rest.
- It is essential to reduce the intake of caffeine, alcohol, and other substances that may disrupt sleep or worsen stress levels.

6. Seek Professional Help When Needed:

- Recognize the signs of burnout, compassion fatigue, or mental health concerns and seek support from mental health professionals if necessary.
- To access confidential support and resources, you can use employee assistance programs (EAPs) or counseling services offered by your workplace.

7. Engage in Activities That Bring Joy and Fulfillment:

- It's important to set aside time for hobbies, interests, and activities to provide happiness, calmness, and satisfaction unrelated to work.
- To nurture your emotional well-being, engage in creative pursuits, spend time in nature, or connect with loved ones.

Taking care of ourselves and our well-being is crucial, particularly for those in high-stress professions like emergency nursing. By prioritizing self-care, implementing stress-management techniques, fostering supportive relationships, setting boundaries, and practicing healthy lifestyle habits, we can maintain our resilience and cope with the challenges that come our way. In addition, it's also essential to seek help from qualified professionals and engage in activities that bring us joy and satisfaction. By prioritizing our well-being, we can remain healthy and happy.

Case Studies and Scenarios

Incorporating case studies and scenarios into emergency nursing education reinforces key concepts and allows learners to apply theoretical knowledge to real-world situations. Here are a few examples:

Case Study 1:

Scenario:

In the emergency department, a man of 45 years old has complained of chest pain. He describes the pain as crushing and radiating to his left arm. He appears diaphoretic and anxious.

Case Study Questions:

1. What initial actions should the nurse take upon receiving this patient?
2. What assessments are crucial in determining the severity of the patient's condition?
3. What differential diagnoses should be considered based on the patient's symptoms?
4. How should the nurse prioritize care for this patient, considering the potential diagnosis of myocardial infarction (MI)?

5. What interventions should be implemented to manage the patient's chest pain and stabilize his condition?

Case Study 2:

Scenario:

In the emergency department, a woman who was 30 years old arrived with a deep laceration on her forearm, which she sustained while cooking. The wound is bleeding profusely, and the patient appears pale and dizzy.

Case Study Questions:

1. What immediate actions should the nurse take to manage the patient's bleeding?
2. How should the nurse assess the severity of the laceration and the need for further intervention?
3. What supplies and equipment are required for wound care and hemostasis?
4. How should the nurse prioritize care for this patient, considering the potential for hypovolemic shock?
5. What instructions should be provided to the patient for wound care and follow-up?

Case Study 3:

Scenario:

A male patient, aged 65, arrives at the emergency department presenting with difficulty in breathing and a productive cough that expels mucus. The individual has a history of COPD and is a smoker.

Case Study Questions:

1. What initial assessments should the nurse perform to evaluate the patient's respiratory status?
2. How should the nurse prioritize care for this patient, considering his history of COPD and acute exacerbation of symptoms?
3. What interventions should improve the patient's oxygenation and respiratory function?
4. What pharmacological treatments may be indicated for managing COPD exacerbation?
5. How should the nurse educate the patient on self-management strategies and follow-up care?

Incorporating case studies and scenarios into emergency nursing education can enhance learners' engagement with the material, improve critical thinking skills, and get practical experience in assessing and managing various patient presentations. These real-world examples help bridge the gap between theory and practice, ultimately boosting the competency and confidence of emergency nurses.

8

Conclusion

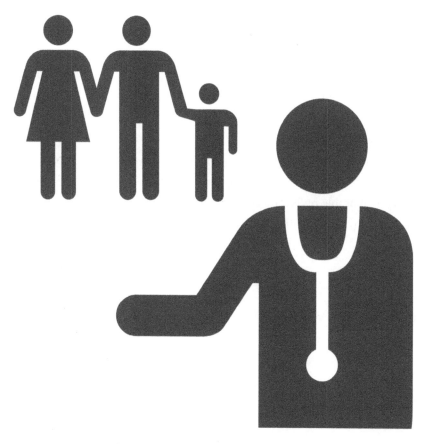

Congratulations on completing the thrilling journey through 'Emergency Nursing Made Simple'! This book is not just your average read; it's a game-changer for your professional growth and a roadmap to excellence in emergency nursing. The book has delved into essential skills, strategies, and techniques that will empower you to provide top-notch patient care and take your practice to the next level. Emergency nursing is not just a job; it's a calling, and you are a beacon of hope and healing in times of crisis.

As you continue your journey, remember that you are making an extraordinary impact on the lives of those you serve. Your curiosity, compassion, and commitment to lifelong learning and growth make you an exceptional emergency nurse. Thank you for joining me on this adventure. You are the unsung heroes of the ER, and together, we can make a difference in our patients' lives, one step at a time!

We appreciate your interest in this book and are thrilled to have you join us. Let's streamline emergency nursing practices and inspire others to embrace this exciting field! If you found this book helpful, please leave a favorable review on Amazon. Your review will encourage others to join us in this thrilling journey of emergency nursing!

9

References

AdventHealth Home. (2022, April 29). *Code Stroke: The ER is the first place to go when stroke symptoms strike.* AdventHealth. https://www.adventhealth.com/business/adventhealth-central-florida-media-resources/news/code-stroke-er-first-place-go-when-stroke-symptoms-strike

Bsn, T. U., RN. (2023, January 2). 10 Important qualities of a good ER nurse - Nurse money talk. *Nurse Money Talk.* https://nursemoneytalk.com/blog/qualities-of-a-good-er-nurse

Gauer, R., Forbes, D., & Boyer, N. (2020, April 1). *Sepsis: Diagnosis and management.* AAFP. https://www.aafp.org/pubs/afp/issues/2020/0401/p409.html https://www.acep.org/patient-care/policy-statements/standardized-protocols-for-optimizing-emergency-department-care/

Msn, K. K., RN. (2023, April 21). Head-to-Toe Nursing Assessments versus Focused Assessments – FRESHRN. *Head-to-Toe Nursing Assessments versus Focused Assessments.* Retrieved March 9, 2024, from

https://www.freshrn.com/nursing-assessments-head-to-toe-versus-fo
cused-assessments/.

Quinn, P.T. (2009) 'The evolving role of the Patient Advocate in the emergency department: The experience of one community hospital,' *Journal
of Emergency Nursing*, 35(1), pp. 48–49. doi:10.1016/j.jen.2007.06.023.

Slypher, T. (2023) *The 10 rights of Medication Administration, Vivian
Community Hub*.Available at: https://www.vivian.com/community/he
althcare-education/medication-administration/ (Accessed: 09 March
2024).

Standardized protocols for optimizing emergency department care. (n.d.).
ACEP.org. https://www.acep.org/patient-care/policy-statements/stan
dardized-protocols-for-optimizing-emergency-department-care/

Stettler, H. (no date b) *800-424-4888 | www.ttuhsc.edu/health.edu 1 a
January 9, 2015 report ...,https://healthedu.ttuhsc.edu/applicationfiles/Ed
uFiles/Text/314121.manuscript.pdf.* Available at: https://www.ttuhsc
.edu/LMS/LMSSupportFiles/EduFiles/Text/80117.manuscript.pdf
(Accessed: 10 March 2024).

Torrey, T. (2024b) *What Medical Triage is and how it is used to prioritize
treatment, VerywellHealth.* Available at: https://www.verywellhealth.co
m/medical-triage-and-how-it-works-2615132 (Accessed: 09 March
2024).

What does an ER nurse do? (2023) *CareerExplorer.* Available at:https://w
ww.careerexplorer.com/careers/er-nurse/ (Accessed: 09 March 2024).

Writers, S. (2023, February 10). How to become an ER nurse |

NurseJournal.org. *NurseJournal.* https://nursejournal.org/careers/
er-nurse/how-to-become/

Yancey, C. C., & O'Rourke, M. C. (2023, August 28). *Emergency
department triage.* StatPearls - NCBI Bookshelf. https://www.ncbi.
nlm.nih.gov/books/NBK557583/

WebMD Editorial Contributors. (2011, April 23). *What is a code blue?*
WebMD. https://www.webmd.com/a-to-z-guides/what-is-a-code-blu
e

Zamberg, I., Mtsweni, N., & Staff, C. (2023, December 21). *Standardizing
ER protocols and Procedures: Consistency in crisis.* C8 Health. https://c8h
ealth.com/a/blog/standardizing-er-protocols-and-procedures-consist
ency-in-crisis

Made in United States
Cleveland, OH
16 July 2025

18598917R00046